Transforming Fluff to Fitness:

Unlocking the Path to Total Wellness and Sustainable Fitness

By

Dr. Elizabeth H. Frazier

Transforming Fluff to Fitness

Copyright © by Dr. Elizabeth H. Frazier 2023. All rights reserved.

TABLE OF CONTENTS

Transforming Fluff to Fitness

Introduction

Welcome to the book "Transforming Fluff to Fitness: Unlocking the Path to Total Wellness and Sustainable Fitness." This book is a map that will lead you on a revolutionary journey to a better, fitter, and more rewarding existence.

This book seeks to reinvent the concept of fitness in a world that frequently promotes appearance over wellbeing. It's not just about losing weight or sculpting muscles; it's about taking a comprehensive approach to health that includes physical, mental, and emotional wellbeing. It is a journey that everyone willing to accept may go on, not only professional athletes or fitness specialists.

The transition from "fluff" to "fitness" is more than just a physical transformation; it also involves a significant change in lifestyle, mindset, and behaviours. It's about making long-term adjustments that lead to better health, more vitality, and a revitalized sense of self-assurance.

Transforming Fluff to Fitness

Throughout these pages, you'll find insights, methods, and actionable steps to help you on your path to improved health. This book is your entire guide to everything from understanding the value of balanced nutrition to creating efficient training routines and from cultivating a positive mindset to forming sustainable habits.

We'll look at the concepts of mindful eating, the value of varying workout regimens, and the role of mental resilience in reaching fitness objectives. Each chapter is designed to give you valuable skills and knowledge that you can apply in your daily life.

We will work together to solve any difficulties or problems that may occur along the way.

On the path from "fluff" to "fitness," there is hope for a happier, healthier future. Imagine waking up to a vibrant life, beginning each day with a cheerful attitude, and confidently fulfilling your objectives. You will feel better about your physical and emotional health and have more energy. It is about reclaiming life in its totality, not just beauty.

Numerous people's experiences on this route attest to the fact that transformation is hugely satisfying and feasible.

Transforming Fluff to Fitness

Personal growth and physical fitness are both necessary components of this journey.

This book is a companion on your journey to holistic wellness, not merely a blueprint for physical transformation. "Transforming Fluff to Fitness" is here to assist and guide you, whether you're a beginner taking your first steps toward fitness or someone looking to rejuvenate their health journey.

Before we proceed, I'd like you to pause for a moment to reflect. Consider yourself more active, fit, and alive in the future. It is not a pipe dream; it is a reality.

You can make it a reality.

Make a vow to yourself and this trip that you will take the first step toward being the healthy, active, and confident version of yourself.

This is when the transformation from "fluff" to "fitness" begins. Let's dive in together and discover the path to comprehensive wellbeing and long-term fitness.

Chapter 1

Understanding Your Current Way of Life

All it takes is becoming intensely aware of your current habits, health, and way of life.

Examining Your Current Lifestyle and Health Habits

Before you can begin your journey to fitness, you must first understand your current state. Take some time to assess your performance. Consider your daily routine and overall wellbeing.

Ask yourself the following questions:

1. How physically fit are you at the moment?

2. What is your usual eating routine? Are the foods you consume healthful and well-balanced?

3. How do you feel on a daily basis, both physically and mentally?

Keep a journal to help you with this self-evaluation. Keep track of your daily activities, food and beverage preferences, and energy levels in a diary.

Transforming Fluff to Fitness

These will provide you with a clear image of your current lifestyle and assist you in identifying areas that need to change.

Recognizing the Problem

After you've examined your health and activities, it's time to focus on the issue areas. These are the things in your life that could be keeping you from being happy. Perhaps you've become sedentary or have poor eating habits. Identifying these areas is an essential first step toward positive change.

Identifying the Problem(s)

Why did you form your current habits and lifestyle? Examine the root causes of your conduct.

Common qualities that contribute to unhealthy lifestyles include:

1. Limited time
2. Eating for psychological reasons
3. Excessive anxiety
4. Time constraints at work

Understanding the underlying causes can allow you to address them more effectively while you attempt to lose weight.

Transforming Fluff to Fitness

The Emotional Connection to Health

Your physical and mental wellbeing are inextricably intertwined. Stress, emotional eating, and low self-esteem can all be detrimental to your overall health. Recognize the emotional ties that exist between your health and your lifestyle choices. This information will help you make better decisions and deal with the moving parts of your journey.

Having Reasonable Expectations

Setting reasonable expectations is essential for this transition. Recognize that there is no one-size-fits-all or quick-fix answer for this trip. It's a steady and sluggish process. You're making long-term life adjustments. Establish reasonable expectations and schedules to achieve success and minimize disappointment.

The Value of Reflection

Finally, remember the need for self-compassion. Avoid self-criticism and self-blame. Compassion for oneself is a transforming solid catalyst. Be as gentle and sympathetic

Transforming Fluff to Fitness

with yourself as you would with a friend going through a similar situation.

Willingness to adapt

Decide to follow your transformational path. Consider this surgery an investment in your future health. The road ahead is full of exciting adventures, but it may also contain some problems. Accepting self-compassion and comprehending your current way of life is a significant first step toward long-term change.

Chapter 2

What you need to know about fitness and weight loss to succeed

Success in fitness and weight loss requires education, commitment, and constant work.

SET SMART AND ATTAINABLE OBJECTIVES:

For your fitness and fat loss objectives, set specific, measurable, and time-bound exercises. A clear goal will keep you focused and motivated.

- **Recognize Nutrition:** A healthy diet is essential for fat loss. Consume healthful foods such as lean proteins, complex carbohydrates, healthy fats, and fruits and vegetables.

- If you want to lose weight, keep track of your calorie intake and make sure you're in a caloric deficit.

Transforming Fluff to Fitness

- **Keep hydrated:** Drink enough water to improve your metabolism and general wellness. Dehydration may impair fat loss.
- **Exercise on a regular basis:** Include aerobic (such as jogging or cycling) and strength training (such as weightlifting) workouts in your program.

- **Strength exercise** has been shown to increase metabolism and stimulate muscular growth.
- **The Key to Consistency:** The critical aspect of fat loss is consistency. Maintain your long-term exercise and nutrition strategy.
- **Reduce Stress:** Stress might cause overeating, making fat reduction more difficult. Use stress-reduction strategies such as yoga, meditation, and deep breathing.
- **Get Enough Sleep:** Sleep deprivation can influence hunger and appetite hormones. Attempt to get eight or nine hours of quality sleep each night.
- **Track Your Progress:** You can keep track of your progress using fitness software or a journal. Keep track of your nutrition, physical activity, and any changes in body composition.

Transforming Fluff to Fitness

- **Fad diets should be avoided:** Avoid extreme diets that promise quick results. They are frequently unsustainable and may be damaging to your health.
- **Be patient:** losing fat takes time. Don't let sluggish progress discourage you. Prioritize long-term success over short-term remedies.

- **Consult an Expert:** To develop a tailored strategy, consider working with a skilled fitness trainer or nutritionist.
- **Maintain a good mindset:** In order to achieve, you must maintain a good mood. Maintain your good attitude and enjoy your small achievements.
- **Seek Help:** Talk to people who have similar interests as you. Having others witness your journey might help you stay accountable and inspired.
- **Change Your Strategy:** Keep an open mind to fresh ideas. As your body evolves, your plan may need to adapt.

Keep in mind that there is no one-size-fits-all solution to weight loss and fitness. What works well for you might not work best for someone else. Tailor your plan to your unique needs and preferences for long-term success, and most importantly, make it a sustainable part of your lifestyle.

Chapter 3

Food, Delicious Meal

The phrase "Food, Delicious Meal" usually conjures up images of joy and festivity associated with eating meals. It refers to how important food is to our survival.

Food serves a number of essential functions.

1. Nutrition: Food is the primary source of essential vitamins, minerals, and nutrients that our bodies require to function correctly. A healthy diet supports overall health.

2. Importance in Culture: Food is inextricably linked to customs and festivities. Ancestry, traditions, or familial relationships can all be represented by it.

Transforming Fluff to Fitness

3. Sensual pleasure: Food smells, scents, textures, and colors all contribute to a sensory experience that can be immensely gratifying and pleasurable.

4. Social Connection: Sharing meals with loved ones strengthens bonds and provides opportunities for engagement and dialogue.

5. Comfort and Emotional Support: During challenging circumstances, food can provide both emotional and physical support.

6. Creativity: Cooking is a popular way for people to express themselves artistically. Experimenting with ingredients and trying new meals may be fun and exciting.

7. Health and Happiness: A nutrient-dense, well-balanced diet can help manage or avoid medical disorders, improving long-term health and wellbeing.

Finally, food is more than just a source of nourishment; it is a vital part of who we are, influencing our emotional, cultural, and physical wellbeing.

Food and Nutrition

A healthy diet is essential for moving from "fluff" to "fitness."

Transforming Fluff to Fitness

This chapter delves deeply into the principles of diet and nutrition, assisting you in learning how to fuel your body for fat loss and overall health.

Nutrition in Moderation

Any successful fitness and weight loss journey begins with a well-balanced diet. It comprises consuming a variety of foods that have nutrients that enhance overall health and wellbeing.

What you should understand:

1. Macronutrients: The three primary macronutrients that should be included in your diet are carbohydrates, proteins, and fats. Carbohydrates give energy, proteins aid in muscle growth and repair, and healthy fats are required for a variety of biological functions.

2. Micronutrients are vitamins and minerals that your body needs in small amounts yet are necessary for optimal health. Make sure that your food is healthy.

3. Hydration: Water is a necessary nutrient. Staying hydrated boosts metabolism, aids in hunger regulation, and aids in meal digestion and absorption.

Transforming Fluff to Fitness

Calorie Intake and Fat Loss

A calorie deficit is essential for fat loss success. It entails consuming fewer calories than you burn.

How to Monitor Your Calorie Intake

- **Energy Requirements:** Calculate your daily maintenance calories (TDEE - Total Daily Energy Expenditure) to learn how many calories you need to maintain your current weight.

- **Caloric Deficiency:** To lose fat, create a slight caloric deficit, usually around 500 calories per day. It can result in a progressive and sustainable 1-pound-per-week weight decrease.

- **Calorie Counting:** Keep a meal journal or use an app to keep track of your calorie intake. It allows you to stay inside your calorie budget.

Meal Planning and Portion Control

A balanced diet necessitates good meal planning and portion control:

Transforming Fluff to Fitness

- **Routine of Meals**: Regular, well-balanced meals might help you control your metabolism and avoid overeating.
- **Portion Sizes:** Pay attention to portion proportions to avoid overconsumption. To help with portion management, use smaller plates.

Healthy Food Alternatives

Make healthy eating choices by focusing on whole, unprocessed foods.

- **Low-fat proteins:** Include lean meats, chicken, fish, tofu, and beans in your diet for muscle repair and growth.
- **Complex Carbohydrates:** Choose whole grains, vegetables, and fruits as your primary carbohydrate sources for long-lasting energy.
- **Healthy Fats:** Avocados, almonds, seeds, and olive oil are all excellent sources of essential fatty acids.

Transforming Fluff to Fitness

Avoiding Common Errors

1. Processed Foods: Avoid processed and fast foods that are heavy in added sugars, unhealthy fats, and empty calories.

2. Mindful Eating: Practice mindful eating by observing hunger and fullness cues and savoring the tastes of your food.

Dietary Change

Diversify your diet to ensure you get a wide range of nutrients:

1. Colourful Plate: A colorful plate typically signifies a wide range of nutrients. To make your meals more colorful, include a variety of fruits and vegetables.

2. Rotation: Change your meals to minimize dietary monotony and to ensure you are getting a diverse range of nutrients.

How to Calculate Macros

Transforming Fluff to Fitness

Calculating your macronutrients (macronutrients) is the process of determining the right combination of carbohydrates, proteins, and fats in your diet to fulfill your specific fitness and health goals.

A simple approach for calculating macros

Determine Your Goals:

Do you want to lose weight, add muscle, or maintain your current weight? Your goal will determine your macro ratios.

Calculating Total Daily Energy Expenditure (TDEE):

Use an online TDEE calculator or see a fitness consultant to determine your daily calorie needs. TDEE considers your BMR and level of activity.

Calorie Distribution among Macros: The way your macronutrients are determined is determined by your daily calorie intake.

The general guidelines are as follows:

1. Proteins: Protein should make up 10-35% of your daily calorie intake. A typical target range is 15-25%.

2. Carbohydrates: Carbohydrates should account for 45-65% of your total daily calorie intake. 45-55% is a typical target range.

Transforming Fluff to Fitness

3. Fats: Fats should comprise 20-35% of your daily calorie intake. A typical target range is 20-30%.

Calorie to Gram Conversion: Protein and carbohydrates have four calories per gram, while fat contains nine calories per gram. Convert the calories supplied to each macro into grams using these calculations. If you wish to take 20% of your daily calories from fat and your TDEE is 2,000 calories, you would do the following:
(0.20 x 2,000) / 9 = 44 g fat

Depending on Your Goal, Make the Following Changes: If you want to lose weight, aim for a little higher protein intake to maintain lean muscle mass. If you're going to gain muscle, you should consume more carbohydrates.

Keep an eye on your macros:
To ensure you are meeting your daily macronutrient objectives, keep a meal journal, utilize a nutrition app, or see a dietitian. Keeping track of your food consumption will assist you in staying on track.

Transforming Fluff to Fitness

Calorie Calculation

Calculating your daily calorie needs is an essential step in nutrition management, regardless of whether your goal is weight reduction, maintenance, or growth. There are several methods for calculating your daily calorie intake.

A straightforward technique for calculating your daily calorie intake.

Determine Your Basal Metabolic Rate (BMR): Your BMR is the number of calories your body requires at rest to perform essential functions such as breathing and circulation. The Harris-Benedict equation is one of several formulas that may be used to calculate your BMR.

The following are the formulas for calculating your BMR:

BMR = 88.362 + (13.397 x weight in kg) + (4.799 x height in cm) - (5.677 x age in years) for men

BMR = 447.593 + (9.247 x weight in kg) + (3.098 x height in cm) - (4.330 x age in years) for women

Consider your level of activity (TDEE – Total Daily Energy Expenditure):

Transforming Fluff to Fitness

The calories burned during normal activity and exercise are factored into your TDEE.

Your activity level is classified as follows:

Sedentary (no or little physical activity): BMR x 1.2

Lightly active (1-3 days of light exercise or sports per week): BMR x 1.375

Moderately active (3-5 days of moderate exercise or sports per week): BMR x 1.55

Very Active (6-7 days of intense training or sports per week): BMR x 1.725

If you are Active (perform a lot of intense exercises or have physically demanding work and exercise twice a day), multiply your BMR by 1.9.

Determine Your Goals

Determine whether you want to lose, maintain, or gain weight. As needed, adjust your daily calorie intake:

1. To lose weight, consume fewer calories than your TDEE, resulting in a caloric deficit. A 500-calorie deficit each day is recommended, resulting in a weekly loss of about 1 pound.

Transforming Fluff to Fitness

2. Consume calories equivalent to your TDEE to maintain your present weight.

3. Create a caloric surplus by eating more calories than your TDEE, often with an additional 250-500 calories per day for sustained weight gain.

Maintain and modify

Maintain a diary of your calorie consumption and progress. Depending on how your goals and outcomes change over time, you may need to tweak your calorie intake.

Keep in mind that these are simply estimates and that individual variations exist. It is better to obtain personalized guidance from a licensed dietitian or nutritionist based on your specific needs, goals, and health problems. They can help you create a precise and tailored food plan.

Chapter 4

Handling Sugar Cravings

Transforming Fluff to Fitness

Although controlling sugar cravings can be difficult, there are a few strategies you can employ to prevent and minimize them:

Many Strategies for Handling and Reducing Sugar Cravings

1. Remain Hydrated: Sometimes, desires for sugar or hunger can be mistaken for thirst. Drink enough water to stay hydrated all day.

2. Eat Frequently: Skipping meals can alter blood sugar levels, which may lead to cravings. Aim for regular, well-balanced meals and snacks.

3. Choose Whole Foods: Pick complete, unprocessed foods. Healthy fats, lean proteins, and whole grains can all help control blood sugar levels and prevent cravings.

4. Macros Must Be Balanced: Make sure your meals have a balance of macronutrients (fats, proteins, and carbohydrates) to help reduce cravings. Healthy fats and protein are incredibly satisfying.

5. Incorporate Fiber: Eating a diet rich in fruits, vegetables, and whole grains will help you feel full and content and reduce your desire for certain foods.

Transforming Fluff to Fitness

6. Arrange Your Meals and Snacks: Prepare wholesome meals and snacks in advance. Keeping healthy options close at hand might reduce the likelihood of making rash, poor choices.

7. Cut Down on Added Sugars: Pay attention to any additional sugars in your diet. Choose foods with less added sugar by reading food labels to find hidden sugar sources.

8. Eating with Intention: Pay attention to the food you're consuming. Savor the tastes and textures of your cuisine. Overeating and cravings can be lessened with mindful eating.

9. Control Your Stress: Cravings may result from too much stress. Mindfulness, yoga, and deep breathing are all techniques for lowering pressure.

10. Get Enough Sleep: Hormones that control appetite and hunger can be disrupted by sleep deprivation. Make an effort to get 8 or 9 hours of sound sleep each night.

11. Exercise: Getting regular exercise can reduce cravings and help control blood sugar levels. Even a short stroll can be helpful.

Transforming Fluff to Fitness

12. Keep yourself occupied: Engaging in hobbies or activities can assist in diverting your focus from cravings. Look for a helpful way to pass the time.

13. Make healthier substitutions: Fresh fruit, yogurt with honey, or dark chocolate with a high cocoa content are good options if you're craving something sweet.

14. Exercise Moderation: It is okay to overindulge if you have a sweet craving occasionally. Here, moderation is a key term. Scoop up a tiny bit and enjoy the taste.

15. Seek Assistance: For specialized guidance and techniques, consider consulting with a licensed dietitian or nutritionist if you experience intense sugar cravings.

Recall that desires for sugar are typical and that they occur frequently. The way you handle and react to such urges is what counts. By making better decisions and putting these strategies into practice, you can lessen the intensity and frequency of your sugar cravings and work toward a more gratifying and balanced diet.

Chapter 5

Exercise and Fitness

Working out is crucial to making the transition from "fluff" to "fitness." This chapter explores the critical impact that fitness and exercise play in changing your appearance and overall health.

Types of Exercise

A well-rounded fitness regimen must include a variety of exercises:

1. Cardiovascular Exercise: Exercises that increase heart rate, burn calories, and improve cardiovascular health include swimming, cycling, and jogging. They are excellent at burning fat.

2. Strengthening Activities: Strength training, which usually involves resistance training or weight lifting, improves muscle growth, speeds up metabolism, and results in a more defined and toned physique.

3. Flexibility and mobility: exercises that increase joint mobility, reduce the chance of injury, and improve balance include yoga and stretching regimens.

Transforming Fluff to Fitness

4. Functional Training: By enhancing everyday activities and boosting general strength and endurance, practical exercises, including bodyweight workouts and efficient motions, are beneficial.

Creating a Schedule for Exercise
The following elements need to be carefully taken into account when designing a fitness program that works:
1. Establishing Goals: Establish your fitness goals, including increased endurance, muscle growth, and weight loss. Your goals will determine your training program.
2. Frequency: Choose how often you are going to work out. Aim for at least 150 minutes per week of moderate-intensity aerobic exercise or 75 minutes per week of vigorous-intensity aerobic exercise, per health standards.
3. Duration: Choose how long you want to work out. It would help if you mixed up the length of your workouts by incorporating more extended endurance-building activities with shorter, high-intensity sessions.

Transforming Fluff to Fitness

4. Intensity: It's essential to consider the intensity level. Your routines should incorporate both lower-intensity, steady-state cardio and high-intensity interval training (HIIT).

5. Strengthening Exercises: it's recommended to engage in strength training two to three times a week, focusing on various muscle groups to build and tone your body.

Change and advancement

Sustained success necessitates ongoing development.

- **Progressive Overload:** Gradually up the weight, duration, or intensity of your workouts to challenge your body and promote growth.
- **Variety:** Mix a range of exercises, routines, and activities to keep workouts interesting and prevent plateaus.

Motivation and Attitude

Motivation and an optimistic outlook are essential for staying on course.

1. Establish realistic expectations: Understand that change is a process. Small triumphs need to be celebrated, and steady progress shouldn't be discouraged.

Transforming Fluff to Fitness

2. Preserve Accountability: Tell a friend about your fitness objectives or ask a workout partner for assistance. Accountability may make people more motivated.

3. Monitor Your Development: Use wearables, notebooks, or fitness apps to track your progress and see how far you've come.

4. Relaxation and Healing: Allow your body to get the rest it needs:

5. Vacation days: Regularly schedule rest days to prevent burnout and to give your body time to heal and repair. Establishing priorities for sleep is crucial since it's necessary for general wellbeing and muscle repair.

Chapter 6

Motivation and Steadiness

It will need motivation and perseverance to go from "fluff" to "fitness." This chapter covers the essential elements of maintaining consistency in your efforts and being driven to reach your fitness goals.

Motivational Comprehending

The inner need that propels you to action is known as motivation. In order to maintain motivation:

1. Establish clear goals: Clearly define your fitness goals. Having dreams will keep you motivated, whether they are for increased endurance, muscular building, or weight loss.

2. Intrinsic Motivation: Find out what drives you from within. Long-term motivation can be sustained by tying your fitness journey to your goals and values.

3. Outside Insight: Make use of external motivational resources like accolades, words of support from loved ones, or accountability partners.

Transforming Fluff to Fitness

4. Envision Success: To envision success, picture what you want to happen in your mind's eye. This goal has the potential to be a powerful motivator.

5. Monitor Your Development: Regularly assess and celebrate your achievements. Maintaining a record of your advancement makes you feel accomplished.

6. Adjust Your Goals: In order to continue on your journey, you should adjust and set new goals when you reach your previous ones.

Maintaining Uniformity

The secret to long-term success is consistency.

1. Exercise regimen: Establish a regimen that turns into a habit. Maintaining consistency helps your body change and evolve with time.

2. Accountability: Talk to a fitness coach or your workout partner about your objectives so they can help you stay on track.

3. Planning: Schedule your meals and exercise in advance. Making snap decisions is less likely when you have a plan in place.

Transforming Fluff to Fitness

4. Flexibility: Be flexible even if you must stick to a routine. Because life can be unpredictable, it's a good idea to adjust as necessary without losing hope.

5. Social Support: Assemble a group of friends or similar fitness enthusiasts who are supportive of your goals.

6. Positive Reinforcement: Give yourself something nice for being reliable. Celebrate the victories and significant junctures you've reached.

7. Overcoming Difficulties: Difficulties are a natural part of the journey. Keep moving forward, make any required adjustments to your plan, and ask for help as needed.

Keeping Up Your Motivation Despite Adversity

Acknowledge that challenges and setbacks are unavoidable

Accept Failure: In order to succeed, one must first overcome failure. Please take what you've learned from your errors and apply it to your next endeavors.

Modify Your Objectives: It's okay to adjust your aims or strategy if you run across problems.

Because the road is not straight, flexibility is needed.

Transforming Fluff to Fitness

Mind resilience: Build mental toughness to help you get through challenging circumstances. Positivity and self-compassion are incredible traits.

Chapter 7

Successful Meal Planning

Organizing your meals is a great way to accomplish your health and fitness objectives. In order to make eating a healthy, balanced diet easier, it involves prepping your meals and snacks.

How to properly organize your meals

1. Set Specific Goals: Decide on your dietary objectives, such as improved general health, muscle building, or weight loss. Your aims will guide your meal preparation decisions.

2. Create a Meal Plan: List breakfast, lunch, dinner, and snacks for each week. Make sure a lot of fruits, vegetables, complex carbohydrates, lean proteins, and healthy fats are included in your meals.

3. Create a Shopping List: To make sure you have all the supplies, create a thorough shopping list based on your meal plan. Follow your inventory to prevent impulsive purchases.

4. Choose a Prep Day: Every week, set aside a particular day to prepare meals. Many individuals find that Sunday works well, so pick a day that works for you.

5. Cook in Bulk: Prepare dishes in bulk so you can eat the leftovers for several days. It reduces the need to cook every day and saves time.

6. Make an Investment in Containers: Purchase a variety of meal prep containers in different sizes to accommodate other meal portions. These containers ought to be dishwasher and microwave-safe for convenience.

7. Portion Control: Use meal prep containers to portion your meals based on your dietary objectives. It helps you maintain your routine and prevents overeating.

8. Label and Date: Label every container with the name of the product and the date it was produced. It ensures that meals are eaten before they go bad.

9. Variety and Taste: To keep your diners interested, use a variety of tastes and components in your meal preparation. Try a variety of foods and flavors to prevent boredom.

Transforming Fluff to Fitness

10. Provide Snacks: To stave off hunger in between meals, whip up some nutritious snacks like mixed nuts or chopped fruits and veggies.

11. Freeze Meals: Consider freezing some of the meals you prepare ahead of time to keep them fresh throughout the week.

12. Maintain Organization: Store all of your prepared meals in a freezer or refrigerator that is conveniently accessible to help you stay organized when preparing meals.

13. Be Adaptable: You don't have to follow a set recipe when preparing meals. Be flexible and adjust your meal plans to account for any last-minute schedule adjustments or social obligations.

14. Clean as You Go: Wash dishes and utensils while you prepare meals and afterward. It facilitates supervision of the cleanup process.

Not only does meal planning save you time, but it also enables you to choose healthier options rather than relying on bad takeout or convenience meals.

Transforming Fluff to Fitness

By organizing and cooking your meals in advance, you position yourself for success in your search for good health and a balanced diet.

Chapter 8

Alcohol and Fat Loss

Alcohol usage can hinder fat loss and overall health. Understanding its effects is crucial for anyone embarking on a fitness or weight loss journey

Impact of Alcohol in the Body

1. Empty Calories: Alcohol has seven calories per gram, making it more calorie-rich than carbs and protein. Drinking alcohol can raise your calorie intake dramatically and, if ignored, could impair your efforts to shed fat.

2. Slows Metabolism: Alcohol can interfere with your body's metabolism by lowering the rate at which you burn calories. It can have an impact on your capacity to drop weight.

Transforming Fluff to Fitness

3. Increased hunger: Alcohol can stimulate appetite and weaken inhibitions, leading to overeating or making inappropriate food choices when drinking. Excess calorie consumption can inhibit fat decrease.

4. Modifies Macronutrient Processing: The body favors alcohol metabolism above lipids, proteins, and carbohydrates. When alcohol accumulates in your system, your body prioritizes digestion, potentially storing these other macronutrients as fat.

5. Reduces Inhibitions: Alcohol can affect your self-control and judgment, causing you to consume less carefully and possibly overindulge in high-calorie, unhealthy foods.

6. Dehydration: Because alcohol is a diuretic, it can cause dehydration. Dehydrated cells metabolize fat less efficiently, making it more challenging to burn stored fat.

7. Sleep: Alcohol can disrupt sleep patterns, lowering the quality and quantity of sleep. Sleep deprivation could create hormonal imbalances that limit fat reduction.

Transforming Fluff to Fitness

8. Effect on Workout Recovery: Excessive alcohol consumption can hinder your ability to recover from workouts and lower training performance.

9. Liver Function: The liver processes alcohol, and heavy drinking can lead it to become stressed, decreasing its ability to metabolize fats adequately.

10. Depletion of Nutrients: Alcohol can deplete critical vitamins and minerals, such as B vitamins and magnesium that are essential for overall health and energy metabolism.

Moderation and Balance

If you like to drink alcohol while working toward fat loss and fitness objectives, moderation is vital.

Guidelines on Moderation and Balance

1. Limit your alcohol intake and be conscious of the calories it contributes to your diet

2. Select lower-calorie alcoholic beverages such as light beer, wine, or spirits with calorie-free mixers.

3. Drink plenty of water before, during, and after ingesting alcohol to stay hydrated.

Transforming Fluff to Fitness

4. Avoid binge drinking and overindulging, especially when accompanied by poor nutritional choices.
Plan your alcohol usage properly, taking into account the timing of your exercises and meals.
5. Monitor the influence of alcohol on your development and, if required, adjust your consumption.

Finally, alcohol and fat reduction can coexist if you are careful of your usage and make suitable changes to your diet and lifestyle. Balancing your fitness goals with social or personal drinking decisions is feasible with a planned and informed approach.

Chapter 9

How to Manage Pain and Discomfort

Managing pain and discomfort, especially after vigorous exercise, is crucial for overall health and injury prevention.

Ideas on how to handle pain and soreness effectively

1. Rest and recovery: Allow your body time to heal after an intense workout. It's usual for discomfort to accompany your muscles' natural healing and growing processes.

2. Stretching: Include gentle stretching exercises in your routine, focusing on the sore muscles. Stretching can aid

Transforming Fluff to Fitness

in the alleviation of muscle tension and the enhancement of flexibility.

3. Foam Rolling: A foam roller is attainable to accomplish self-myofascial relaxation. Rolling out tight places can help reduce muscle tension and discomfort.

4. Hydration: Stay hydrated at all times. Dehydration can increase muscle pains and cramps.

5. Nutrition: To minimize inflammation, consume a well-balanced diet high in protein and anti-inflammatory foods such as berries, fatty salmon, and leafy greens.

6. Over-the-counter pain medicines: Non-prescription pain medicines such as ibuprofen or acetaminophen can provide brief relief. Use them as prescribed, and seek the counsel of a healthcare specialist if you have any concerns.

7. Heat and ice: In the first 48 hours following strenuous exercise, apply ice to decrease inflammation. Heat can then aid in releasing stiff muscles and increase blood flow.

Transforming Fluff to Fitness

8. Massage: To reduce muscle stress and discomfort, try getting a professional massage or using a massage tool.

9. Epsom Salt Bath: Soaking in an Epsom salt bath can help relax muscles and reduce stiffness.

10. Active recovery entails engaging in light physical exercise such as walking or swimming. It can enhance blood flow and aid in healing.

11. Quality Sleep: Make sure you receive enough of it. Sleep is crucial for muscle regeneration and pain alleviation.

12. Warm-up and cool-down properly: Always warm up before the exercise and cool down afterward. It can aid in injury prevention and minimize post-workout soreness.

13. Pay Attention to Your Body: If you are suffering sharp or severe pain that does not improve with self-care, you should seek medical attention. Pain might be an indicator of an underlying condition that requires expert attention.

Transforming Fluff to Fitness

Remember that some soreness is typical, particularly if you push your body during workouts. However, it's vital to find a balance between exerting oneself and avoiding overexertion, which can result in terrible pain and even injury.

Chapter 10

Maintaining Your Progress

Your shift from Fluff to fitness is a continual process that does not cease after you attain your original fitness goals. This chapter focuses on how to maintain your success while building a long-term, sustainable attitude toward health and fitness.

Transforming Fluff to Fitness

Sustainability and Way of Life

Integrating health and exercise into your routine is the key to preserving your progress.

How to go about it

1. Mindset Change: Change your perspective from short-term to long-term. Instead of focusing on instant remedies, prioritize long-term health and wellness.

2. Consistency: Maintain the behaviors and routines that helped you reach your initial goals. The foundation of long-term progress is consistency.

3. Flexibility: As your requirements and circumstances change, be adaptive and open to changes in your exercise and food choices.

4. Moderation: It is vital when it comes to diet and exercise. To reduce exhaustion and frustration, strive for a balanced approach.

5. Pay Attention to Your Body's Messages: Pay attention to your body's messages. Rest when necessary, change your workouts and adjust your nutrition when essential.

6. Set New Objectives: Set fresh exercise goals to keep your trip enjoyable. It can be related to strength,

Transforming Fluff to Fitness

endurance, or even recreational activities such as racing or participation in events.

7. Intuitive Eating: Rather than following severe dietary rules, intuitive eating emphasizes listening to your body's hunger and fullness sensations. It can assist you in keeping your success without the limits of diets.

Essential components of intuitive eating

1. Mindful Eating: It requires paying attention to what you eat and relishing the flavors and textures of your food. These can assist you in making better-balanced selections.

2. Hunger Control: Eat when you are hungry and quit when you are full. Eat not out of boredom or emotion.

3. No Guilt or Shame: Don't equate guilt or shame with your eating choices. All foods, in small amounts, can be part of a balanced diet.

4. Enjoyment: Prioritizing foods you enjoy can help you maintain a healthy eating pattern.

Transforming Fluff to Fitness

5.   Social   and   environmental   support: Your surroundings and social ties can have a significant impact on your potential to succeed.

6. Social Support: Maintain contact with friends and family who share your fitness and health goals. Consider training companions or fitness sessions with a social component.

7. Wellness Atmosphere: Create a healthy environment that helps your goals, such as keeping nutritious foods at home.

8. Reflection and Evaluation: It is vital to reflect on your travel and analyze your development often.

9. Journaling: Keep a journal to track your fitness and nutrition and even to document your bodily and emotional health.

10. Enjoy Success: To stay motivated and appreciate your hard work, enjoy your minor and significant accomplishments.

11. Establish checkpoints: Assess your progress often to verify you are on track and make any necessary modifications.

Transforming Fluff to Fitness

Conclusion

As we come to the end of "Transforming Fluff to Fitness: Unlocking the Path to Total Wellness and Sustainable

Transforming Fluff to Fitness

Fitness," it's not just the end of a book but the start of a new chapter in your quest to a better, more fulfilled life.

Throughout these pages, we've looked at the many facets of wellness, delving into diet, exercise, mindset, and sustainability. This book's goal was not merely to deliver information but also to spark a transformation within you, one based on conscious decisions, balanced practices, and an unrelenting commitment to your wellbeing.

Remember that your fitness journey is a marathon, not a sprint—one that requires patience, perseverance, and self-kindness. Every step, no matter how tiny, is a step closer to a healthier you.

As you finish this chapter, keep the ideas of balanced nutrition, varied fitness regimens, and a good outlook in mind. Accept the pleasure of fueling your body with nutritious foods, savor the energy of energizing workouts, and build a mindset that values progress over perfection.

Your wellness journey is continuing, and the lessons you've learned here are stepping stones that will lead you to long-term health and pleasure. You can turn obstacles into opportunities and failures into victories.

Transforming Fluff to Fitness

Allow the ideas contained in this book to guide you on your journey to total wellness. Embrace the road, savor every victory, big or small and keep pushing forward because proper fitness is a way of life, not a destination.

Thank you for being a part of this life-changing adventure. May your journey to comprehensive wellness and long-term fitness be filled with strength, vitality, and a strong sense of accomplishment.

I wish you great success and a life full of health and vitality.

Continue to be inspired, maintain your dedication, and maintain your fitness.